My Health & Fitness Goals

I0415267

Goal One

Goal	
Motivation	
Reward	

Goal Two

Goal	
Motivation	
Reward	

Goal Three

Goal	
Motivation	
Reward	

Weekly Health & Fitness Tracker

Week of:_____

Sleep Goal:_____

Hydration Goal:_____

Calories Goal:_____

My Motivation

My Exercise Goal This Week

My Health Goal This Week

Words for When I Need a Motivation Boost

Exercise Log

	Goal	Actual
Mon		
Tues		
Wed		
Thurs		
Fri		
Sat		
Sun		

Positive thought:_____

Health Log			
	Sleep (hrs)	Water intake	Calorie intake
Mon			
Tues			
Wed			
Thurs			
Fri			
Sat			
Sun			

What Went Well?

Healthy Habits							
Habit	M	T	W	T	F	S	S

Could Go Better

Next Week Will Bring

Daily Plan & Tracker

Date:_____

Sleep: ◯◯◯◯◯◯◯◯

Water: ◯◯◯◯◯◯◯◯

Resting HR:_____

Today I feel

Wake up time:

Meal Plan

Breakfast	◯
	◯
	◯
Lunch	◯
	◯
	◯
Dinner	◯
	◯
	◯
Snacks	◯
	◯
	◯

I am motivated because

Stuck to meal plan? ☐

Stuck to exercise plan? ☐

Calorie intake

I am:_____

Exercise Plan

Activity	Time	Sets	Reps	Dist.	
					❑
					❑
					❑
					❑
					❑

Healthy & Happy Tasks

❑
❑
❑
❑
❑
❑
❑

Shopping List

❑
❑
❑
❑
❑

Today's 3 Positives

○
○
○

Notes

Today's Step Count

Bed Time:

Daily Plan & Tracker

Date:_____

Sleep: ○○○○○○○

Water: ○○○○○○○

Resting HR:_____

Today I feel

Wake up time:

Meal Plan

Breakfast	○ ○ ○
Lunch	○ ○ ○
Dinner	○ ○ ○
Snacks	○ ○ ○

I am motivated because

Stuck to meal plan? ☐

Stuck to exercise plan? ☐

Calorie intake

I am:_____

Exercise Plan

Activity	Time	Sets	Reps	Dist.	
					❑
					❑
					❑
					❑
					❑

Healthy & Happy Tasks

❑
❑
❑
❑
❑
❑
❑

Shopping List

❑
❑
❑
❑
❑

Today's 3 Positives

○
○
○

Notes

Today's Step Count

Bed Time:

Daily Plan & Tracker

Date:_____

Sleep: ○○○○○○○○

Water: ○○○○○○○○

Resting HR:_____

Today I feel

Wake up time:

Meal Plan

Breakfast	○ ○ ○
Lunch	○ ○ ○
Dinner	○ ○ ○
Snacks	○ ○ ○

I am motivated because

Stuck to meal plan? ☐

Stuck to exercise plan? ☐

Calorie intake

I am:_____

Exercise Plan					
Activity	Time	Sets	Reps	Dist.	
					❑
					❑
					❑
					❑
					❑

Healthy & Happy Tasks

❑
❑
❑
❑
❑
❑
❑

Shopping List

❑
❑
❑
❑
❑

Today's 3 Positives

○
○
○

Notes

Today's Step Count

Bed Time:

Daily Plan & Tracker

Date:_____

Sleep: ○○○○○○○○

Water: ○○○○○○○○

Resting HR:_____

Today I feel

Wake up time:

Meal Plan

Breakfast	○ ○ ○
Lunch	○ ○ ○
Dinner	○ ○ ○
Snacks	○ ○ ○

I am motivated because

Stuck to meal plan? ☐

Stuck to exercise plan? ☐

Calorie intake

I am:_____

Exercise Plan

Activity	Time	Sets	Reps	Dist.	
					❑
					❑
					❑
					❑
					❑

Healthy & Happy Tasks

❑
❑
❑
❑
❑
❑
❑

Shopping List

❑
❑
❑
❑
❑

Today's 3 Positives

○
○
○

Notes

Today's Step Count

Bed Time:

Daily Plan & Tracker

Date:_____

Sleep: ⭕⭕⭕⭕⭕⭕⭕

Water: ⭕⭕⭕⭕⭕⭕⭕

Resting HR:_____

Today I feel

Wake up time:

Meal Plan	
Breakfast	○ ○ ○
Lunch	○ ○ ○
Dinner	○ ○ ○
Snacks	○ ○ ○

I am motivated because

Stuck to meal plan? ☐

Stuck to exercise plan? ☐

Calorie intake

I am:_____

Exercise Plan

Activity	Time	Sets	Reps	Dist.	
					❑
					❑
					❑
					❑
					❑

Healthy & Happy Tasks

❑
❑
❑
❑
❑
❑
❑

Shopping List

❑
❑
❑
❑
❑

Today's 3 Positives

○
○
○

Notes

Today's Step Count

Bed Time:

Daily Plan & Tracker

Date:_____

Sleep: ◯◯◯◯◯◯◯◯

Water: ◯◯◯◯◯◯◯◯

Resting HR:_____

Today I feel

Wake up time:

Meal Plan

Breakfast	○
	○
	○
Lunch	○
	○
	○
Dinner	○
	○
	○
Snacks	○
	○
	○

I am motivated because

Stuck to meal plan? ☐

Stuck to exercise plan? ☐

Calorie intake

I am:_____

Exercise Plan					
Activity	Time	Sets	Reps	Dist.	
					❑
					❑
					❑
					❑
					❑

Healthy & Happy Tasks

❑
❑
❑
❑
❑
❑
❑

Shopping List

❑
❑
❑
❑
❑

Today's 3 Positives

○
○
○

Notes

Today's Step Count

Bed Time:

Daily Plan & Tracker

Date:_____

Sleep: ○○○○○○○○

Water: ○○○○○○○○

Resting HR:_____

Today I feel

Wake up time:

Meal Plan

Breakfast	○ ○ ○
Lunch	○ ○ ○
Dinner	○ ○ ○
Snacks	○ ○ ○

I am motivated because

Stuck to meal plan? ☐

Stuck to exercise plan? ☐

Calorie intake

I am:_____

Exercise Plan

Activity	Time	Sets	Reps	Dist.	
					❑
					❑
					❑
					❑
					❑

Healthy & Happy Tasks

❑
❑
❑
❑
❑
❑
❑

Shopping List

❑
❑
❑
❑
❑

Today's 3 Positives

○
○
○

Notes

Today's Step Count

Bed Time:

Weekly Health & Fitness Tracker

Week of:_____

Sleep Goal:_____

Hydration Goal:_____

Calories Goal:_____

My Motivation

My Exercise Goal This Week

My Health Goal This Week

Words for When I Need a Motivation Boost

Exercise Log

	Goal	Actual
Mon		
Tues		
Wed		
Thurs		
Fri		
Sat		
Sun		

Positive thought:_____

Health Log			
	Sleep (hrs)	Water intake	Calorie intake
Mon			
Tues			
Wed			
Thurs			
Fri			
Sat			
Sun			

What Went Well?

Healthy Habits

Habit	M	T	W	T	F	S	S

Could Go Better

Next Week Will Bring

Daily Plan & Tracker

Date:_____

Sleep: ⭕⭕⭕⭕⭕⭕⭕

Water: ⭕⭕⭕⭕⭕⭕⭕

Resting HR:_____

Today I feel

Wake up time:

Meal Plan

Breakfast	⭕ ⭕ ⭕
Lunch	⭕ ⭕ ⭕
Dinner	⭕ ⭕ ⭕
Snacks	⭕ ⭕ ⭕

I am motivated because

Stuck to meal plan? ☐

Stuck to exercise plan? ☐

Calorie intake

I am:_____

Exercise Plan

Activity	Time	Sets	Reps	Dist.	
					☐
					☐
					☐
					☐
					☐

Healthy & Happy Tasks

☐
☐
☐
☐
☐
☐
☐

Shopping List

☐
☐
☐
☐
☐

Today's 3 Positives

○
○
○

Notes

Today's Step Count

Bed Time:

Daily Plan & Tracker

Date:_____

Sleep: ○○○○○○○○

Water: ○○○○○○○○

Resting HR:_____

Today I feel

Wake up time:

Meal Plan	
Breakfast	○ ○ ○
Lunch	○ ○ ○
Dinner	○ ○ ○
Snacks	○ ○ ○

I am motivated because

Stuck to meal plan? ☐

Stuck to exercise plan? ☐

Calorie intake

I am:_____

Exercise Plan					
Activity	Time	Sets	Reps	Dist.	
					❑
					❑
					❑
					❑
					❑

Healthy & Happy Tasks

❑
❑
❑
❑
❑
❑
❑

Shopping List

❑
❑
❑
❑
❑

Today's 3 Positives

○
○
○

Notes

Today's Step Count

Bed Time:

Daily Plan & Tracker

Date:_____

Sleep: ○○○○○○○○

Water: ○○○○○○○○

Resting HR:_____

Today I feel

Wake up time:

Meal Plan

Breakfast	○
	○
	○
Lunch	○
	○
	○
Dinner	○
	○
	○
Snacks	○
	○
	○

I am motivated because

Stuck to meal plan? ☐

Stuck to exercise plan? ☐

Calorie intake

I am:_____

Exercise Plan					
Activity	Time	Sets	Reps	Dist.	
					❑
					❑
					❑
					❑
					❑

Healthy & Happy Tasks

❑
❑
❑
❑
❑
❑
❑

Shopping List

❑
❑
❑
❑
❑

Today's 3 Positives

○
○
○

Notes

Today's Step Count

Bed Time:

Daily Plan & Tracker

Date:_____

Sleep: ◯◯◯◯◯◯◯◯

Water: ◯◯◯◯◯◯◯◯

Resting HR:_____

Today I feel

Wake up time:

Meal Plan

Breakfast	◯
	◯
	◯

Lunch	◯
	◯
	◯

Dinner	◯
	◯
	◯

Snacks	◯
	◯
	◯

I am motivated because

Stuck to meal plan? ☐

Stuck to exercise plan? ☐

Calorie intake

I am:_____

Exercise Plan

Activity	Time	Sets	Reps	Dist.	
					☐
					☐
					☐
					☐
					☐

Healthy & Happy Tasks

☐
☐
☐
☐
☐
☐
☐

Shopping List

☐
☐
☐
☐
☐

Today's 3 Positives

○
○
○

Notes

Today's Step Count

Bed Time:

Daily Plan & Tracker

Date:_____

Sleep: ⭕⭕⭕⭕⭕⭕⭕

Water: ⭕⭕⭕⭕⭕⭕⭕

Resting HR:_____

Today I feel

Wake up time:

Meal Plan

Breakfast	○ ○ ○
Lunch	○ ○ ○
Dinner	○ ○ ○
Snacks	○ ○ ○

I am motivated because

Stuck to meal plan? ☐

Stuck to exercise plan? ☐

Calorie intake

I am:_____

Exercise Plan					
Activity	Time	Sets	Reps	Dist.	
					❑
					❑
					❑
					❑
					❑

Healthy & Happy Tasks

❑
❑
❑
❑
❑
❑
❑

Shopping List

❑
❑
❑
❑
❑

Today's 3 Positives

○
○
○

Notes

Today's Step Count

Bed Time:

Daily Plan & Tracker

Date:_____

Sleep: ○○○○○○○○

Water: ○○○○○○○○

Resting HR:_____

Today I feel

Wake up time:

Meal Plan

Breakfast	○ ○ ○
Lunch	○ ○ ○
Dinner	○ ○ ○
Snacks	○ ○ ○

I am motivated because

Stuck to meal plan? ☐

Stuck to exercise plan? ☐

Calorie intake

I am:_____

Exercise Plan

Activity	Time	Sets	Reps	Dist.	
					❑
					❑
					❑
					❑
					❑

Healthy & Happy Tasks

❑
❑
❑
❑
❑
❑
❑

Shopping List

❑
❑
❑
❑
❑

Today's 3 Positives

○
○
○

Notes

Bed Time:

Today's Step Count

Daily Plan & Tracker

Date:_____

Sleep: ○○○○○○○○

Water: ○○○○○○○○

Resting HR:_____

Today I feel

Wake up time:

Meal Plan

Breakfast	○ ○ ○
Lunch	○ ○ ○
Dinner	○ ○ ○
Snacks	○ ○ ○

I am motivated because

Stuck to meal plan? ☐

Stuck to exercise plan? ☐

Calorie intake

I am:_____

Exercise Plan

Activity	Time	Sets	Reps	Dist.	
					❏
					❏
					❏
					❏
					❏

Healthy & Happy Tasks

❏
❏
❏
❏
❏
❏
❏

Shopping List

❏
❏
❏
❏
❏

Today's 3 Positives

○
○
○

Notes

Today's Step Count

Bed Time:

Weekly Health & Fitness Tracker

Week of:_____

Sleep Goal:_____
Hydration Goal:_____
Calories Goal:_____

My Motivation

My Exercise Goal This Week

My Health Goal This Week

Words for When I Need a Motivation Boost

Exercise Log

	Goal	Actual
Mon		
Tues		
Wed		
Thurs		
Fri		
Sat		
Sun		

Positive thought:_____

Health Log

	Sleep (hrs)	Water intake	Calorie intake
Mon			
Tues			
Wed			
Thurs			
Fri			
Sat			
Sun			

What Went Well?

Healthy Habits

Habit	M	T	W	T	F	S	S

Could Go Better

Next Week Will Bring

Daily Plan & Tracker

Date:_____

Sleep: ⭕⭕⭕⭕⭕⭕⭕⭕

Water: ⭕⭕⭕⭕⭕⭕⭕⭕

Resting HR:_____

Today I feel

Wake up time:

Meal Plan

Breakfast	○ ○ ○
Lunch	○ ○ ○
Dinner	○ ○ ○
Snacks	○ ○ ○

I am motivated because

Stuck to meal plan? ☐

Stuck to exercise plan? ☐

Calorie intake

I am:_____

Exercise Plan

Activity	Time	Sets	Reps	Dist.	
					❑
					❑
					❑
					❑
					❑

Healthy & Happy Tasks

❑
❑
❑
❑
❑
❑
❑

Shopping List

❑
❑
❑
❑
❑

Today's 3 Positives

○
○
○

Notes

Today's Step Count

Bed Time:

Daily Plan & Tracker

Date:_____

Sleep: ○○○○○○○○

Water: ○○○○○○○○

Resting HR:_____

Today I feel

Wake up time: [   ]

Meal Plan

Breakfast	○
	○
	○
Lunch	○
	○
	○
Dinner	○
	○
	○
Snacks	○
	○
	○

I am motivated because

Stuck to meal plan? [ ]
Stuck to exercise plan? [ ]

Calorie intake

I am:_____

Exercise Plan					
Activity	Time	Sets	Reps	Dist.	
					❑
					❑
					❑
					❑
					❑

Healthy & Happy Tasks

❑
❑
❑
❑
❑
❑
❑

Shopping List

❑
❑
❑
❑
❑

Today's 3 Positives

○
○
○

Notes

Today's Step Count

Bed Time:

Daily Plan & Tracker

Date:_____

Sleep: ◯◯◯◯◯◯◯◯

Water: ◯◯◯◯◯◯◯◯

Resting HR:_____

Today I feel

Wake up time:

Meal Plan

Breakfast	◯
	◯
	◯
Lunch	◯
	◯
	◯
Dinner	◯
	◯
	◯
Snacks	◯
	◯
	◯

I am motivated because

Stuck to meal plan? ☐

Stuck to exercise plan? ☐

Calorie intake

I am:_____

Exercise Plan					
Activity	Time	Sets	Reps	Dist.	
					❑
					❑
					❑
					❑
					❑

Healthy & Happy Tasks

❑
❑
❑
❑
❑
❑
❑

Shopping List

❑
❑
❑
❑
❑

Today's 3 Positives

○
○
○

Notes

Today's Step Count

Bed Time:

Daily Plan & Tracker

Date:_____

Sleep: ○○○○○○○○

Water: ○○○○○○○○

Resting HR:_____

Today I feel

Wake up time:

Meal Plan

Breakfast	○
	○
	○

Lunch	○
	○
	○

Dinner	○
	○
	○

Snacks	○
	○
	○

I am motivated because

Stuck to meal plan? ☐

Stuck to exercise plan? ☐

Calorie intake

I am:_____

Exercise Plan					
Activity	Time	Sets	Reps	Dist.	
					❑
					❑
					❑
					❑
					❑

Healthy & Happy Tasks

❑
❑
❑
❑
❑
❑
❑

Shopping List

❑
❑
❑
❑
❑

Today's 3 Positives

○
○
○

Notes

Today's Step Count

Bed Time:

Daily Plan & Tracker

Date:_____

Sleep: ○○○○○○○○

Water: ○○○○○○○○

Resting HR:_____

Today I feel

Wake up time:

Meal Plan

Breakfast	○
	○
	○

Lunch	○
	○
	○

Dinner	○
	○
	○

Snacks	○
	○
	○

I am motivated because

Stuck to meal plan? ☐
Stuck to exercise plan? ☐

Calorie intake

I am:_____

Exercise Plan

Activity	Time	Sets	Reps	Dist.	
					☐
					☐
					☐
					☐
					☐

Healthy & Happy Tasks

☐
☐
☐
☐
☐
☐
☐

Shopping List

☐
☐
☐
☐
☐

Today's 3 Positives

○
○
○

Notes

Today's Step Count

Bed Time:

Daily Plan & Tracker

Date:_____

Sleep: ○○○○○○○○

Water: ○○○○○○○○

Resting HR:_____

Today I feel

Wake up time:

Meal Plan

Breakfast	○
	○
	○
Lunch	○
	○
	○
Dinner	○
	○
	○
Snacks	○
	○
	○

I am motivated because

Stuck to meal plan? ☐

Stuck to exercise plan? ☐

Calorie intake

I am:_____

Exercise Plan					
Activity	Time	Sets	Reps	Dist.	
					❑
					❑
					❑
					❑
					❑

Healthy & Happy Tasks

- ❑
- ❑
- ❑
- ❑
- ❑
- ❑
- ❑

Shopping List

- ❑
- ❑
- ❑
- ❑
- ❑

Today's 3 Positives

- ○
- ○
- ○

Notes

Today's Step Count

Bed Time:

Daily Plan & Tracker

Date:_____

Sleep: ◯◯◯◯◯◯◯◯

Water: ◯◯◯◯◯◯◯◯

Resting HR:_____

Today I feel

Wake up time:

Meal Plan	
Breakfast	◯ ◯ ◯
Lunch	◯ ◯ ◯
Dinner	◯ ◯ ◯
Snacks	◯ ◯ ◯

I am motivated because

Stuck to meal plan? ☐

Stuck to exercise plan? ☐

Calorie intake

I am:_____

Exercise Plan

Activity	Time	Sets	Reps	Dist.	
					❑
					❑
					❑
					❑
					❑

Healthy & Happy Tasks

❑
❑
❑
❑
❑
❑
❑

Shopping List

❑
❑
❑
❑
❑

Today's 3 Positives

○
○
○

Notes

Today's Step Count

Bed Time:

Weekly Health & Fitness Tracker

Week of:_____

Sleep Goal:_____

Hydration Goal:_____

Calories Goal:_____

My Motivation

My Exercise Goal This Week

My Health Goal This Week

Words for When I Need a Motivation Boost

Exercise Log

	Goal	Actual
Mon		
Tues		
Wed		
Thurs		
Fri		
Sat		
Sun		

Positive thought:_____

Health Log			
	Sleep (hrs)	Water intake	Calorie intake
Mon			
Tues			
Wed			
Thurs			
Fri			
Sat			
Sun			

What Went Well?

Healthy Habits

Habit	M	T	W	T	F	S	S

Could Go Better

Next Week Will Bring

Daily Plan & Tracker

Date:_____

Sleep: ⬭⬭⬭⬭⬭⬭⬭

Water: ⬭⬭⬭⬭⬭⬭⬭

Resting HR:_____

Today I feel

Wake up time: _____

Meal Plan

Breakfast	○ ○ ○
Lunch	○ ○ ○
Dinner	○ ○ ○
Snacks	○ ○ ○

I am motivated because

Stuck to meal plan? ☐

Stuck to exercise plan? ☐

Calorie intake

I am:_____

Exercise Plan					
Activity	Time	Sets	Reps	Dist.	
					☐
					☐
					☐
					☐
					☐

Healthy & Happy Tasks

☐
☐
☐
☐
☐
☐
☐

Shopping List

☐
☐
☐
☐
☐

Today's 3 Positives

○
○
○

Notes

Today's Step Count

Bed Time:

Daily Plan & Tracker

Date:_____

Sleep: ◯◯◯◯◯◯◯◯

Water: ◯◯◯◯◯◯◯◯

Resting HR:_____

Today I feel

Wake up time:

Meal Plan

Breakfast	◯ ◯ ◯
Lunch	◯ ◯ ◯
Dinner	◯ ◯ ◯
Snacks	◯ ◯ ◯

I am motivated because

Stuck to meal plan? ☐

Stuck to exercise plan? ☐

Calorie intake

I am:_____

Exercise Plan					
Activity	Time	Sets	Reps	Dist.	
					❏
					❏
					❏
					❏
					❏

Healthy & Happy Tasks

❏
❏
❏
❏
❏
❏
❏

Shopping List

❏
❏
❏
❏
❏

Today's 3 Positives

○
○
○

Notes

Today's Step Count

Bed Time:

Daily Plan & Tracker

Date:_____

Sleep: ○○○○○○○○

Water: ○○○○○○○○

Resting HR:_____

Today I feel

Wake up time:

Meal Plan

Breakfast	○ ○ ○
Lunch	○ ○ ○
Dinner	○ ○ ○
Snacks	○ ○ ○

I am motivated because

Stuck to meal plan? ☐

Stuck to exercise plan? ☐

Calorie intake

I am:_____

Exercise Plan

Activity	Time	Sets	Reps	Dist.	
					☐
					☐
					☐
					☐
					☐

Healthy & Happy Tasks

☐
☐
☐
☐
☐
☐
☐

Shopping List

☐
☐
☐
☐
☐

Today's 3 Positives

○
○
○

Notes

Today's Step Count

Bed Time:

Daily Plan & Tracker

Date:_____

Sleep: ⬯⬯⬯⬯⬯⬯⬯⬯

Water: ⬯⬯⬯⬯⬯⬯⬯⬯

Resting HR:_____

Today I feel

Wake up time:

Meal Plan

Breakfast	○ ○ ○
Lunch	○ ○ ○
Dinner	○ ○ ○
Snacks	○ ○ ○

I am motivated because

Stuck to meal plan? ☐

Stuck to exercise plan? ☐

Calorie intake

I am:_____

Exercise Plan					
Activity	Time	Sets	Reps	Dist.	
					❑
					❑
					❑
					❑
					❑

Healthy & Happy Tasks
❑
❑
❑
❑
❑
❑
❑

Shopping List
❑
❑
❑
❑
❑

Today's 3 Positives
○
○
○

Notes

Today's Step Count

Bed Time:

Daily Plan & Tracker

Date:_____

Sleep: ○○○○○○○○

Water: ○○○○○○○○

Resting HR:_____

Today I feel

Wake up time:

Meal Plan

Breakfast	○ ○ ○
Lunch	○ ○ ○
Dinner	○ ○ ○
Snacks	○ ○ ○

I am motivated because

Stuck to meal plan? ☐

Stuck to exercise plan? ☐

Calorie intake

I am:_____

Exercise Plan

Activity	Time	Sets	Reps	Dist.	
					❑
					❑
					❑
					❑
					❑

Healthy & Happy Tasks

❑
❑
❑
❑
❑
❑
❑

Shopping List

❑
❑
❑
❑
❑

Today's 3 Positives

○
○
○

Notes

Today's Step Count

Bed Time:

Daily Plan & Tracker

Date:_____

Sleep: ○○○○○○○○

Water: ○○○○○○○○

Resting HR:_____

Today I feel

Wake up time:

Meal Plan

Breakfast	○ ○ ○
Lunch	○ ○ ○
Dinner	○ ○ ○
Snacks	○ ○ ○

I am motivated because

Stuck to meal plan? ☐

Stuck to exercise plan? ☐

Calorie intake

I am:_____

Exercise Plan

Activity	Time	Sets	Reps	Dist.	
					☐
					☐
					☐
					☐
					☐

Healthy & Happy Tasks

☐
☐
☐
☐
☐
☐
☐

Shopping List

☐
☐
☐
☐
☐

Today's 3 Positives

○
○
○

Notes

Today's Step Count

Bed Time:

Daily Plan & Tracker

Date:_____

Sleep: ⬭⬭⬭⬭⬭⬭⬭

Water: ⬭⬭⬭⬭⬭⬭⬭

Resting HR:_____

Today I feel

Wake up time:

Meal Plan

Breakfast	○
	○
	○
Lunch	○
	○
	○
Dinner	○
	○
	○
Snacks	○
	○
	○

I am motivated because

Stuck to meal plan? ☐

Stuck to exercise plan? ☐

Calorie intake

I am:_____

Exercise Plan

Activity	Time	Sets	Reps	Dist.	
					❑
					❑
					❑
					❑
					❑

Healthy & Happy Tasks

❑
❑
❑
❑
❑
❑
❑

Shopping List

❑
❑
❑
❑
❑

Today's 3 Positives

○
○
○

Notes

Bed Time:

Today's Step Count

Weekly Health & Fitness Tracker

Week of:_____

Sleep Goal:_____

Hydration Goal:_____

Calories Goal:_____

My Motivation

My Exercise Goal This Week

My Health Goal This Week

Words for When I Need a Motivation Boost

Exercise Log

	Goal	Actual
Mon		
Tues		
Wed		
Thurs		
Fri		
Sat		
Sun		

Positive thought:_____

Health Log			
	Sleep (hrs)	Water intake	Calorie intake
Mon			
Tues			
Wed			
Thurs			
Fri			
Sat			
Sun			

What Went Well?

Healthy Habits

Habit	M	T	W	T	F	S	S

Could Go Better

Next Week Will Bring

Daily Plan & Tracker

Date:_____

Sleep: ⭕⭕⭕⭕⭕⭕⭕⭕

Water: ⭕⭕⭕⭕⭕⭕⭕⭕

Resting HR:_____

Today I feel

Wake up time: [   ]

Meal Plan

Breakfast	○ ○ ○
Lunch	○ ○ ○
Dinner	○ ○ ○
Snacks	○ ○ ○

I am motivated because

Stuck to meal plan? [ ]

Stuck to exercise plan? [ ]

Calorie intake

I am:_____

Exercise Plan

Activity	Time	Sets	Reps	Dist.	
					❑
					❑
					❑
					❑
					❑

Healthy & Happy Tasks

- ❑
- ❑
- ❑
- ❑
- ❑
- ❑
- ❑

Shopping List

- ❑
- ❑
- ❑
- ❑
- ❑

Today's 3 Positives

- ○
- ○
- ○

Notes

Today's Step Count

Bed Time:

Daily Plan & Tracker

Date:_____

Sleep: ⬭⬭⬭⬭⬭⬭⬭⬭

Water: ⬭⬭⬭⬭⬭⬭⬭⬭

Resting HR:_____

Today I feel

Wake up time:

Meal Plan	
Breakfast	○ ○ ○
Lunch	○ ○ ○
Dinner	○ ○ ○
Snacks	○ ○ ○

I am motivated because

Stuck to meal plan? ☐

Stuck to exercise plan? ☐

Calorie intake

I am:_____

Exercise Plan

Activity	Time	Sets	Reps	Dist.	
					❏
					❏
					❏
					❏
					❏

Healthy & Happy Tasks

❏
❏
❏
❏
❏
❏
❏

Shopping List

❏
❏
❏
❏
❏

Today's 3 Positives

○
○
○

Notes

Today's Step Count

Bed Time:

Daily Plan & Tracker

Date:_____

Sleep: ⭕⭕⭕⭕⭕⭕⭕⭕

Water: ⭕⭕⭕⭕⭕⭕⭕⭕

Resting HR:_____

Today I feel

Wake up time:

Meal Plan

Breakfast	◯ ◯ ◯
Lunch	◯ ◯ ◯
Dinner	◯ ◯ ◯
Snacks	◯ ◯ ◯

I am motivated because

Stuck to meal plan? ☐

Stuck to exercise plan? ☐

Calorie intake

I am:_____

Exercise Plan

Activity	Time	Sets	Reps	Dist.	
					❏
					❏
					❏
					❏
					❏

Healthy & Happy Tasks

❏
❏
❏
❏
❏
❏
❏

Shopping List

❏
❏
❏
❏
❏

Today's 3 Positives

○
○
○

Notes

Bed Time:

Today's Step Count

Daily Plan & Tracker

Date:_____

Sleep: ○○○○○○○○

Water: ○○○○○○○○

Resting HR:_____

Today I feel

Wake up time:

Meal Plan

Breakfast	○ ○ ○
Lunch	○ ○ ○
Dinner	○ ○ ○
Snacks	○ ○ ○

I am motivated because

Stuck to meal plan? ☐

Stuck to exercise plan? ☐

Calorie intake

I am:_____

Exercise Plan

Activity	Time	Sets	Reps	Dist.	
					❑
					❑
					❑
					❑
					❑

Healthy & Happy Tasks

❑
❑
❑
❑
❑
❑
❑

Shopping List

❑
❑
❑
❑
❑

Today's 3 Positives

○
○
○

Notes

Today's Step Count

Bed Time:

Daily Plan & Tracker

Date:_____

Sleep: ⚬⚬⚬⚬⚬⚬⚬

Water: ⚬⚬⚬⚬⚬⚬⚬

Resting HR:_____

Today I feel

Wake up time:

Meal Plan	
Breakfast	○ ○ ○
Lunch	○ ○ ○
Dinner	○ ○ ○
Snacks	○ ○ ○

I am motivated because

Stuck to meal plan? ☐

Stuck to exercise plan? ☐

Calorie intake

I am:_____

Exercise Plan

Activity	Time	Sets	Reps	Dist.	
					❑
					❑
					❑
					❑
					❑

Healthy & Happy Tasks

❑
❑
❑
❑
❑
❑
❑

Shopping List

❑
❑
❑
❑
❑

Today's 3 Positives

○
○
○

Notes

Today's Step Count

Bed Time:

Daily Plan & Tracker

Date:_____

Sleep: ○○○○○○○○

Water: ○○○○○○○○

Resting HR:_____

Today I feel

Wake up time:

Meal Plan

Breakfast	○ ○ ○
Lunch	○ ○ ○
Dinner	○ ○ ○
Snacks	○ ○ ○

I am motivated because

Stuck to meal plan? ☐

Stuck to exercise plan? ☐

Calorie intake

I am:_____

Exercise Plan

Activity	Time	Sets	Reps	Dist.	
					❏
					❏
					❏
					❏
					❏

Healthy & Happy Tasks

❏
❏
❏
❏
❏
❏
❏

Shopping List

❏
❏
❏
❏
❏

Today's 3 Positives

○
○
○

Notes

Bed Time:

Today's Step Count

Daily Plan & Tracker

Date:_____

Sleep: ◯◯◯◯◯◯◯

Water: ◯◯◯◯◯◯◯

Resting HR:_____

Today I feel

Wake up time:

Meal Plan

Breakfast	◯
	◯
	◯
Lunch	◯
	◯
	◯
Dinner	◯
	◯
	◯
Snacks	◯
	◯
	◯

I am motivated because

Stuck to meal plan? ☐

Stuck to exercise plan? ☐

Calorie intake

I am:_____

Exercise Plan

Activity	Time	Sets	Reps	Dist.	
					❑
					❑
					❑
					❑
					❑

Healthy & Happy Tasks

❑
❑
❑
❑
❑
❑
❑

Shopping List

❑
❑
❑
❑
❑

Today's 3 Positives

○
○
○

Notes

Today's Step Count

Bed Time:

Weekly Health & Fitness Tracker

Week of:_____

Sleep Goal:_____

Hydration Goal:_____

Calories Goal:_____

My Motivation

My Exercise Goal This Week

My Health Goal This Week

Words for When I Need a Motivation Boost

Exercise Log

	Goal	Actual
Mon		
Tues		
Wed		
Thurs		
Fri		
Sat		
Sun		

Positive thought:_____

_____

Health Log

	Sleep (hrs)	Water intake	Calorie intake
Mon			
Tues			
Wed			
Thurs			
Fri			
Sat			
Sun			

What Went Well?

Healthy Habits

Habit	M	T	W	T	F	S	S

Could Go Better

Next Week Will Bring

Daily Plan & Tracker

Date:_____

Sleep: ⭕⭕⭕⭕⭕⭕⭕⭕

Water: ⭕⭕⭕⭕⭕⭕⭕⭕

Resting HR:_____

Today I feel

Wake up time:

Meal Plan

Breakfast	○ ○ ○
Lunch	○ ○ ○
Dinner	○ ○ ○
Snacks	○ ○ ○

I am motivated because

Stuck to meal plan? ☐

Stuck to exercise plan? ☐

Calorie intake

I am:_____

Exercise Plan					
Activity	Time	Sets	Reps	Dist.	
					❑
					❑
					❑
					❑
					❑

Healthy & Happy Tasks

❑
❑
❑
❑
❑
❑
❑

Shopping List

❑
❑
❑
❑
❑

Today's 3 Positives

○
○
○

Notes

Today's Step Count

Bed Time:

Daily Plan & Tracker

Date:_____

Sleep: ○○○○○○○○

Water: ○○○○○○○○

Resting HR:_____

Today I feel

Wake up time:

Meal Plan

Breakfast	○
	○
	○
Lunch	○
	○
	○
Dinner	○
	○
	○
Snacks	○
	○
	○

I am motivated because

Stuck to meal plan? ☐

Stuck to exercise plan? ☐

Calorie intake

I am:_____

Exercise Plan

Activity	Time	Sets	Reps	Dist.	
					❑
					❑
					❑
					❑
					❑

Healthy & Happy Tasks

❑
❑
❑
❑
❑
❑
❑

Shopping List

❑
❑
❑
❑
❑

Today's 3 Positives

○
○
○

Notes

Today's Step Count

Bed Time:

Daily Plan & Tracker

Date:_____

Sleep: ⭕⭕⭕⭕⭕⭕⭕

Water: ⭕⭕⭕⭕⭕⭕⭕

Resting HR:_____

Today I feel

Wake up time:

Meal Plan

Breakfast	○ ○ ○
Lunch	○ ○ ○
Dinner	○ ○ ○
Snacks	○ ○ ○

I am motivated because

Stuck to meal plan? ☐

Stuck to exercise plan? ☐

Calorie intake

I am:_____

Exercise Plan

Activity	Time	Sets	Reps	Dist.	
					☐
					☐
					☐
					☐
					☐

Healthy & Happy Tasks

☐
☐
☐
☐
☐
☐
☐

Shopping List

☐
☐
☐
☐
☐

Today's 3 Positives

○
○
○

Notes

Today's Step Count

Bed Time:

Daily Plan & Tracker

Date:_____

Sleep: ○○○○○○○○

Water: ○○○○○○○○

Resting HR:_____

Today I feel

Wake up time:

Meal Plan

Breakfast	○
	○
	○

Lunch	○
	○
	○

Dinner	○
	○
	○

Snacks	○
	○
	○

I am motivated because

Stuck to meal plan? ☐

Stuck to exercise plan? ☐

Calorie intake

I am:_____

Exercise Plan

Activity	Time	Sets	Reps	Dist.	
					❏
					❏
					❏
					❏
					❏

Healthy & Happy Tasks

❏
❏
❏
❏
❏
❏
❏

Shopping List

❏
❏
❏
❏
❏

Today's 3 Positives

○
○
○

Notes

Today's Step Count

Bed Time:

Daily Plan & Tracker

Date:_____

Sleep: ⬭⬭⬭⬭⬭⬭⬭

Water: ⬭⬭⬭⬭⬭⬭⬭

Resting HR:_____

Today I feel

Wake up time:

Meal Plan

Breakfast	○
	○
	○
Lunch	○
	○
	○
Dinner	○
	○
	○
Snacks	○
	○
	○

I am motivated because

Stuck to meal plan? ☐

Stuck to exercise plan? ☐

Calorie intake

I am:_____

Exercise Plan					
Activity	Time	Sets	Reps	Dist.	
					❑
					❑
					❑
					❑
					❑

Healthy & Happy Tasks

❑
❑
❑
❑
❑
❑
❑

Shopping List

❑
❑
❑
❑
❑

Today's 3 Positives

○
○
○

Notes

Today's Step Count

Bed Time:

Daily Plan & Tracker

Date:_____

Sleep: ◯◯◯◯◯◯◯◯

Water: ◯◯◯◯◯◯◯◯

Resting HR:_____

Today I feel

Wake up time:

Meal Plan

Breakfast	◯
	◯
	◯
Lunch	◯
	◯
	◯
Dinner	◯
	◯
	◯
Snacks	◯
	◯
	◯

I am motivated because

Stuck to meal plan? ☐

Stuck to exercise plan? ☐

Calorie intake

I am:_____

Exercise Plan

Activity	Time	Sets	Reps	Dist.	
					☐
					☐
					☐
					☐
					☐

Healthy & Happy Tasks

☐
☐
☐
☐
☐
☐
☐

Shopping List

☐
☐
☐
☐
☐

Today's 3 Positives

○
○
○

Notes

Today's Step Count

Bed Time:

Daily Plan & Tracker

Date:_____

Sleep: ⭕⭕⭕⭕⭕⭕⭕

Water: ⭕⭕⭕⭕⭕⭕⭕

Resting HR:_____

Today I feel

Wake up time:

Meal Plan

Breakfast	○ ○ ○
Lunch	○ ○ ○
Dinner	○ ○ ○
Snacks	○ ○ ○

I am motivated because

Stuck to meal plan? ☐

Stuck to exercise plan? ☐

Calorie intake

I am:_____

Exercise Plan

Activity	Time	Sets	Reps	Dist.	
					❏
					❏
					❏
					❏
					❏

Healthy & Happy Tasks

❏
❏
❏
❏
❏
❏
❏

Shopping List

❏
❏
❏
❏
❏

Notes

Today's 3 Positives

○
○
○

Today's Step Count

Bed Time:

Weekly Health & Fitness Tracker

Week of:_____

Sleep Goal:_____

Hydration Goal:_____

Calories Goal:_____

My Motivation

My Exercise Goal This Week

My Health Goal This Week

Words for When I Need a Motivation Boost

Exercise Log

	Goal	Actual
Mon		
Tues		
Wed		
Thurs		
Fri		
Sat		
Sun		

Positive thought:_____

Health Log			
	Sleep (hrs)	Water intake	Calorie intake
Mon			
Tues			
Wed			
Thurs			
Fri			
Sat			
Sun			

What Went Well?

Healthy Habits

Habit	M	T	W	T	F	S	S

Could Go Better

Next Week Will Bring

Daily Plan & Tracker

Date:_____

Sleep: ○○○○○○○○

Water: ○○○○○○○○

Resting HR:_____

Today I feel

Wake up time:

Meal Plan

Breakfast	○ ○ ○
Lunch	○ ○ ○
Dinner	○ ○ ○
Snacks	○ ○ ○

I am motivated because

Stuck to meal plan? ☐

Stuck to exercise plan? ☐

Calorie intake

I am:_____

Exercise Plan

Activity	Time	Sets	Reps	Dist.	
					❑
					❑
					❑
					❑
					❑

Healthy & Happy Tasks

❑
❑
❑
❑
❑
❑
❑

Shopping List

❑
❑
❑
❑
❑

Today's 3 Positives

○
○
○

Notes

Today's Step Count

Bed Time:

Daily Plan & Tracker

Date:_____

Sleep: ⭕⭕⭕⭕⭕⭕⭕

Water: ⭕⭕⭕⭕⭕⭕⭕

Resting HR:_____

Today I feel

Wake up time:

Meal Plan

Breakfast	○ ○ ○
Lunch	○ ○ ○
Dinner	○ ○ ○
Snacks	○ ○ ○

I am motivated because

Stuck to meal plan? ☐

Stuck to exercise plan? ☐

Calorie intake

I am:_____

Exercise Plan

Activity	Time	Sets	Reps	Dist.	
					❏
					❏
					❏
					❏
					❏

Healthy & Happy Tasks

❏
❏
❏
❏
❏
❏
❏

Shopping List

❏
❏
❏
❏
❏

Today's 3 Positives

○
○
○

Notes

Today's Step Count

Bed Time:

Daily Plan & Tracker

Date:_____

Sleep: ○○○○○○○○

Water: ○○○○○○○○

Resting HR:_____

Today I feel

Wake up time:

Meal Plan		
Breakfast	○ ○ ○	
Lunch	○ ○ ○	
Dinner	○ ○ ○	
Snacks	○ ○ ○	

I am motivated because

Stuck to meal plan? ☐

Stuck to exercise plan? ☐

Calorie intake

I am:_____

Exercise Plan					
Activity	Time	Sets	Reps	Dist.	
					❑
					❑
					❑
					❑
					❑

Healthy & Happy Tasks

❑
❑
❑
❑
❑
❑
❑

Shopping List

❑
❑
❑
❑
❑

Today's 3 Positives

○
○
○

Notes

Today's Step Count

Bed Time:

Daily Plan & Tracker

Date:_____

Sleep: ○○○○○○○○

Water: ○○○○○○○○

Resting HR:_____

Today I feel

Wake up time:

Meal Plan

Breakfast	○
	○
	○
Lunch	○
	○
	○
Dinner	○
	○
	○
Snacks	○
	○
	○

I am motivated because

Stuck to meal plan? ☐

Stuck to exercise plan? ☐

Calorie intake

I am:_____

Exercise Plan

Activity	Time	Sets	Reps	Dist.	
					❑
					❑
					❑
					❑
					❑

Healthy & Happy Tasks

❑
❑
❑
❑
❑
❑
❑

Shopping List

❑
❑
❑
❑
❑

Today's 3 Positives

○
○
○

Notes

Today's Step Count

Bed Time:

Daily Plan & Tracker

Date:_____

Sleep: ○○○○○○○○

Water: ○○○○○○○○

Resting HR:_____

Today I feel

Wake up time:

Meal Plan

Breakfast	○
	○
	○
Lunch	○
	○
	○
Dinner	○
	○
	○
Snacks	○
	○
	○

I am motivated because

Stuck to meal plan? ☐

Stuck to exercise plan? ☐

Calorie intake

I am:_____

Exercise Plan					
Activity	Time	Sets	Reps	Dist.	
					❑
					❑
					❑
					❑
					❑

Healthy & Happy Tasks

❑
❑
❑
❑
❑
❑
❑

Shopping List

❑
❑
❑
❑
❑

Today's 3 Positives

○
○
○

Notes

Today's Step Count

Bed Time:

Daily Plan & Tracker

Date:_____

Sleep: ○○○○○○○○

Water: ○○○○○○○○

Resting HR:_____

Today I feel

Wake up time:

Meal Plan

Breakfast	○ ○ ○
Lunch	○ ○ ○
Dinner	○ ○ ○
Snacks	○ ○ ○

I am motivated because

Stuck to meal plan? ☐

Stuck to exercise plan? ☐

Calorie intake

I am:_____

Exercise Plan

Activity	Time	Sets	Reps	Dist.	
					❑
					❑
					❑
					❑
					❑

Healthy & Happy Tasks

❑
❑
❑
❑
❑
❑
❑

Shopping List

❑
❑
❑
❑
❑

Today's 3 Positives

○
○
○

Notes

Today's Step Count

Bed Time:

Daily Plan & Tracker

Date:_____

Sleep: ○○○○○○○○

Water: ○○○○○○○○

Resting HR:_____

Today I feel

Wake up time:

	Meal Plan
Breakfast	○ ○ ○
Lunch	○ ○ ○
Dinner	○ ○ ○
Snacks	○ ○ ○

I am motivated because

Stuck to meal plan? ☐

Stuck to exercise plan? ☐

Calorie intake

I am:_____

Exercise Plan

Activity	Time	Sets	Reps	Dist.	
					❑
					❑
					❑
					❑
					❑

Healthy & Happy Tasks

❑
❑
❑
❑
❑
❑
❑

Shopping List

❑
❑
❑
❑
❑

Today's 3 Positives

○
○
○

Notes

Today's Step Count

Bed Time:

Weekly Health & Fitness Tracker

Week of:_____

Sleep Goal:_____
Hydration Goal:_____
Calories Goal:_____

My Motivation

My Exercise Goal This Week

My Health Goal This Week

Words for When I Need a Motivation Boost

Exercise Log

	Goal	Actual
Mon		
Tues		
Wed		
Thurs		
Fri		
Sat		
Sun		

Positive thought:_____

Health Log			
	Sleep (hrs)	Water intake	Calorie intake
Mon			
Tues			
Wed			
Thurs			
Fri			
Sat			
Sun			

What Went Well?

Healthy Habits							
Habit	M	T	W	T	F	S	S

Could Go Better

Next Week Will Bring

Daily Plan & Tracker

Date:_____

Sleep: ○○○○○○○○

Water: ○○○○○○○○

Resting HR:_____

Today I feel

Wake up time:

Meal Plan

Breakfast	○
	○
	○
Lunch	○
	○
	○
Dinner	○
	○
	○
Snacks	○
	○
	○

I am motivated because

Stuck to meal plan? ☐

Stuck to exercise plan? ☐

Calorie intake

I am: _____

Exercise Plan

Activity	Time	Sets	Reps	Dist.	
					☐
					☐
					☐
					☐
					☐

Healthy & Happy Tasks

☐
☐
☐
☐
☐
☐
☐

Shopping List

☐
☐
☐
☐
☐

Today's 3 Positives

○
○
○

Notes

Today's Step Count

Bed Time:

Daily Plan & Tracker

Date:_____

Sleep: ⬭⬭⬭⬭⬭⬭⬭

Water: ⬭⬭⬭⬭⬭⬭⬭

Resting HR:_____

Today I feel

Wake up time:

Meal Plan

Breakfast	○ ○ ○
Lunch	○ ○ ○
Dinner	○ ○ ○
Snacks	○ ○ ○

I am motivated because

Stuck to meal plan? ☐

Stuck to exercise plan? ☐

Calorie intake

I am:_____

Exercise Plan

Activity	Time	Sets	Reps	Dist.	
					❑
					❑
					❑
					❑
					❑

Healthy & Happy Tasks

❑
❑
❑
❑
❑
❑
❑

Shopping List

❑
❑
❑
❑
❑

Today's 3 Positives

○
○
○

Notes

Today's Step Count

Bed Time:

Daily Plan & Tracker

Date:_____

Sleep: ○○○○○○○○

Water: ○○○○○○○○

Resting HR:_____

Today I feel

Wake up time:

Meal Plan

Breakfast	○
	○
	○
Lunch	○
	○
	○
Dinner	○
	○
	○
Snacks	○
	○
	○

I am motivated because

Stuck to meal plan? ☐

Stuck to exercise plan? ☐

Calorie intake

I am:_____

Exercise Plan

Activity	Time	Sets	Reps	Dist.	
					❑
					❑
					❑
					❑
					❑

Healthy & Happy Tasks

❑
❑
❑
❑
❑
❑
❑

Shopping List

❑
❑
❑
❑
❑

Today's 3 Positives

○
○
○

Notes

Bed Time:

Today's Step Count

Daily Plan & Tracker

Date:_____

Sleep: ⭕⭕⭕⭕⭕⭕⭕

Water: ⭕⭕⭕⭕⭕⭕⭕

Resting HR:_____

Today I feel

Wake up time:

Meal Plan

Breakfast	○ ○ ○
Lunch	○ ○ ○
Dinner	○ ○ ○
Snacks	○ ○ ○

I am motivated because

Stuck to meal plan? ☐

Stuck to exercise plan? ☐

Calorie intake

I am:_____

Exercise Plan					
Activity	Time	Sets	Reps	Dist.	
					❑
					❑
					❑
					❑
					❑

Healthy & Happy Tasks

❑
❑
❑
❑
❑
❑
❑

Shopping List

❑
❑
❑
❑
❑

Today's 3 Positives

○
○
○

Notes

Today's Step Count

Bed Time:

Daily Plan & Tracker

Date:_____

Sleep: ○○○○○○○○

Water: ○○○○○○○○

Resting HR:_____

Today I feel

Wake up time:

Meal Plan

Breakfast	○ ○ ○
Lunch	○ ○ ○
Dinner	○ ○ ○
Snacks	○ ○ ○

I am motivated because

Stuck to meal plan? ☐

Stuck to exercise plan? ☐

Calorie intake

I am:_____

Exercise Plan

Activity	Time	Sets	Reps	Dist.	
					☐
					☐
					☐
					☐
					☐

Healthy & Happy Tasks

☐
☐
☐
☐
☐
☐
☐

Shopping List

☐
☐
☐
☐
☐

Today's 3 Positives

○
○
○

Notes

Today's Step Count

Bed Time:

Daily Plan & Tracker

Date:_____

Sleep: ○○○○○○○○

Water: ○○○○○○○○

Resting HR:_____

Today I feel

Wake up time:

Meal Plan

Breakfast	○
	○
	○
Lunch	○
	○
	○
Dinner	○
	○
	○
Snacks	○
	○
	○

I am motivated because

Stuck to meal plan? ☐

Stuck to exercise plan? ☐

Calorie intake

I am:_____

Exercise Plan					
Activity	Time	Sets	Reps	Dist.	
					❑
					❑
					❑
					❑
					❑

Healthy & Happy Tasks

❑
❑
❑
❑
❑
❑
❑

Shopping List

❑
❑
❑
❑
❑

Today's 3 Positives

○
○
○

Notes

Today's Step Count

Bed Time:

Daily Plan & Tracker

Date:_____

Sleep: ○○○○○○○

Water: ○○○○○○○

Resting HR:_____

Today I feel

Wake up time:

Meal Plan

Breakfast	○ ○ ○
Lunch	○ ○ ○
Dinner	○ ○ ○
Snacks	○ ○ ○

I am motivated because

Stuck to meal plan? ☐

Stuck to exercise plan? ☐

Calorie intake

I am:_____

Exercise Plan					
Activity	Time	Sets	Reps	Dist.	
					☐
					☐
					☐
					☐
					☐

Healthy & Happy Tasks

☐
☐
☐
☐
☐
☐
☐

Shopping List

☐
☐
☐
☐
☐

Today's 3 Positives

○
○
○

Notes

Today's Step Count

Bed Time:

Weekly Health & Fitness Tracker

Week of:_____

Sleep Goal:_____
Hydration Goal:_____
Calories Goal:_____

My Motivation

My Exercise Goal This Week

My Health Goal This Week

Words for When I Need a Motivation Boost

Exercise Log

	Goal	Actual
Mon		
Tues		
Wed		
Thurs		
Fri		
Sat		
Sun		

Positive thought:_____

Health Log

	Sleep (hrs)	Water intake	Calorie intake
Mon			
Tues			
Wed			
Thurs			
Fri			
Sat			
Sun			

What Went Well?

Healthy Habits

Habit	M	T	W	T	F	S	S

Could Go Better

Next Week Will Bring

Daily Plan & Tracker

Date:_____

Sleep: ○○○○○○○○

Water: ○○○○○○○○

Resting HR:_____

Today I feel

Wake up time:

Meal Plan

Breakfast	○
	○
	○
Lunch	○
	○
	○
Dinner	○
	○
	○
Snacks	○
	○
	○

I am motivated because

Stuck to meal plan? ☐

Stuck to exercise plan? ☐

Calorie intake

I am:_____

Exercise Plan					
Activity	Time	Sets	Reps	Dist.	
					❑
					❑
					❑
					❑
					❑

Healthy & Happy Tasks

❑
❑
❑
❑
❑
❑
❑

Shopping List

❑
❑
❑
❑
❑

Today's 3 Positives

○
○
○

Notes

Today's Step Count

Bed Time:

Daily Plan & Tracker

Date:_____

Sleep: ○○○○○○○○

Water: ○○○○○○○○

Resting HR:_____

Today I feel

Wake up time:

Meal Plan

Breakfast	○ ○ ○
Lunch	○ ○ ○
Dinner	○ ○ ○
Snacks	○ ○ ○

I am motivated because

Stuck to meal plan? ☐

Stuck to exercise plan? ☐

Calorie intake

I am:_____

Exercise Plan

Activity	Time	Sets	Reps	Dist.	
					❑
					❑
					❑
					❑
					❑

Healthy & Happy Tasks

❑
❑
❑
❑
❑
❑
❑

Shopping List

❑
❑
❑
❑
❑

Today's 3 Positives

○
○
○

Notes

Today's Step Count

Bed Time:

Daily Plan & Tracker

Date:_____

Sleep: ○○○○○○○○

Water: ○○○○○○○○

Resting HR:_____

Today I feel

Wake up time:

Meal Plan

Breakfast	○ ○ ○
Lunch	○ ○ ○
Dinner	○ ○ ○
Snacks	○ ○ ○

I am motivated because

Stuck to meal plan? ☐

Stuck to exercise plan? ☐

Calorie intake

I am:_____

Exercise Plan

Activity	Time	Sets	Reps	Dist.	
					❑
					❑
					❑
					❑
					❑

Healthy & Happy Tasks

❑
❑
❑
❑
❑
❑
❑

Shopping List

❑
❑
❑
❑
❑

Today's 3 Positives

○
○
○

Notes

Today's Step Count

Bed Time:

Daily Plan & Tracker

Date:_____

Sleep: OOOOOOOO

Water: OOOOOOOO

Resting HR:_____

Today I feel

Wake up time:

Meal Plan

Breakfast	O O O
Lunch	O O O
Dinner	O O O
Snacks	O O O

I am motivated because

Stuck to meal plan? ☐

Stuck to exercise plan? ☐

Calorie intake

I am:_____

Exercise Plan

Activity	Time	Sets	Reps	Dist.	
					❑
					❑
					❑
					❑
					❑

Healthy & Happy Tasks

- ❑
- ❑
- ❑
- ❑
- ❑
- ❑
- ❑

Notes

Bed Time:

Shopping List

- ❑
- ❑
- ❑
- ❑
- ❑

Today's 3 Positives

- ○
- ○
- ○

Today's Step Count

Daily Plan & Tracker

Date:_____

Sleep: ○○○○○○○○

Water: ○○○○○○○○

Resting HR:_____

Today I feel

Wake up time:

Meal Plan

Breakfast	○ ○ ○	
Lunch	○ ○ ○	
Dinner	○ ○ ○	
Snacks	○ ○ ○	

I am motivated because

Stuck to meal plan? ☐

Stuck to exercise plan? ☐

Calorie intake

I am:_____

Exercise Plan

Activity	Time	Sets	Reps	Dist.	
					❑
					❑
					❑
					❑
					❑

Healthy & Happy Tasks

❑
❑
❑
❑
❑
❑
❑

Shopping List

❑
❑
❑
❑
❑

Today's 3 Positives

○
○
○

Notes

Today's Step Count

Bed Time:

Daily Plan & Tracker

Date:_____

Sleep: ⭕⭕⭕⭕⭕⭕⭕

Water: ⭕⭕⭕⭕⭕⭕⭕

Resting HR:_____

Today I feel

Wake up time:

Meal Plan	
Breakfast	○ ___ ○ ___ ○ ___
Lunch	○ ___ ○ ___ ○ ___
Dinner	○ ___ ○ ___ ○ ___
Snacks	○ ___ ○ ___ ○ ___

I am motivated because

Stuck to meal plan? ☐

Stuck to exercise plan? ☐

Calorie intake

I am:_____

Exercise Plan

Activity	Time	Sets	Reps	Dist.	
					❑
					❑
					❑
					❑
					❑

Healthy & Happy Tasks

❑
❑
❑
❑
❑
❑
❑

Shopping List

❑
❑
❑
❑
❑

Today's 3 Positives

○
○
○

Notes

Today's Step Count

Bed Time:

Daily Plan & Tracker

Date:_____

Sleep: ⬭⬭⬭⬭⬭⬭⬭

Water: ⬭⬭⬭⬭⬭⬭⬭

Resting HR:_____

Today I feel

Wake up time:

Meal Plan

Breakfast	○ ○ ○
Lunch	○ ○ ○
Dinner	○ ○ ○
Snacks	○ ○ ○

I am motivated because

Stuck to meal plan? ☐

Stuck to exercise plan? ☐

Calorie intake

I am:_____

Exercise Plan

Activity	Time	Sets	Reps	Dist.	
					❑
					❑
					❑
					❑
					❑

Healthy & Happy Tasks

❑
❑
❑
❑
❑
❑
❑

Shopping List

❑
❑
❑
❑
❑

Today's 3 Positives

○
○
○

Notes

Today's Step Count

Bed Time:

Weekly Health & Fitness Tracker

Week of:_____

Sleep Goal:_____

Hydration Goal:_____

Calories Goal:_____

My Motivation

My Exercise Goal This Week

My Health Goal This Week

Words for When I Need a Motivation Boost

Exercise Log

	Goal	Actual
Mon		
Tues		
Wed		
Thurs		
Fri		
Sat		
Sun		

Positive thought:_____

Health Log

	Sleep (hrs)	Water intake	Calorie intake
Mon			
Tues			
Wed			
Thurs			
Fri			
Sat			
Sun			

What Went Well?

Healthy Habits

Habit	M	T	W	T	F	S	S

Could Go Better

Next Week Will Bring

Daily Plan & Tracker

Date:_____

Sleep: ⭕⭕⭕⭕⭕⭕⭕

Water: ⭕⭕⭕⭕⭕⭕⭕

Resting HR:_____

Today I feel

Wake up time:

Meal Plan

Breakfast	○ ○ ○
Lunch	○ ○ ○
Dinner	○ ○ ○
Snacks	○ ○ ○

I am motivated because

Stuck to meal plan? ☐

Stuck to exercise plan? ☐

Calorie intake

I am:_____

Exercise Plan

Activity	Time	Sets	Reps	Dist.	
					❏
					❏
					❏
					❏
					❏

Healthy & Happy Tasks

❏
❏
❏
❏
❏
❏
❏

Shopping List

❏
❏
❏
❏
❏

Today's 3 Positives

○
○
○

Notes

Today's Step Count

Bed Time:

Daily Plan & Tracker

Date:_____

Sleep: ○○○○○○○○

Water: ○○○○○○○○

Resting HR:_____

Today I feel

Wake up time:

Meal Plan

Breakfast	○ ○ ○
Lunch	○ ○ ○
Dinner	○ ○ ○
Snacks	○ ○ ○

I am motivated because

Stuck to meal plan? ☐

Stuck to exercise plan? ☐

Calorie intake

I am:_____

Exercise Plan

Activity	Time	Sets	Reps	Dist.	
					☐
					☐
					☐
					☐
					☐

Healthy & Happy Tasks

☐
☐
☐
☐
☐
☐
☐

Shopping List

☐
☐
☐
☐
☐

Today's 3 Positives

○
○
○

Notes

Today's Step Count

Bed Time:

Daily Plan & Tracker

Date:_____

Sleep: ○○○○○○○○

Water: ○○○○○○○○

Resting HR:_____

Today I feel

Wake up time:

Meal Plan

Breakfast	○ ○ ○
Lunch	○ ○ ○
Dinner	○ ○ ○
Snacks	○ ○ ○

I am motivated because

Stuck to meal plan? ☐

Stuck to exercise plan? ☐

Calorie intake

I am:_____

Exercise Plan

Activity	Time	Sets	Reps	Dist.	
					❑
					❑
					❑
					❑
					❑

Healthy & Happy Tasks

❑
❑
❑
❑
❑
❑
❑

Shopping List

❑
❑
❑
❑
❑

Today's 3 Positives

○
○
○

Notes

Today's Step Count

Bed Time:

Daily Plan & Tracker

Date:_____

Sleep: ⬭⬭⬭⬭⬭⬭⬭⬭

Water: ⬭⬭⬭⬭⬭⬭⬭⬭

Resting HR:_____

Today I feel

Wake up time:

Meal Plan	
Breakfast	○ ○ ○
Lunch	○ ○ ○
Dinner	○ ○ ○
Snacks	○ ○ ○

I am motivated because

Stuck to meal plan? ☐

Stuck to exercise plan? ☐

Calorie intake

I am:_____

Exercise Plan

Activity	Time	Sets	Reps	Dist.	
					❑
					❑
					❑
					❑
					❑

Healthy & Happy Tasks

❑
❑
❑
❑
❑
❑
❑

Shopping List

❑
❑
❑
❑
❑

Today's 3 Positives

○
○
○

Notes

Today's Step Count

Bed Time:

Daily Plan & Tracker

Date:_____

Sleep: ○○○○○○○○

Water: ○○○○○○○○

Resting HR:_____

Today I feel

Wake up time:

Meal Plan

Breakfast	○ ○ ○
Lunch	○ ○ ○
Dinner	○ ○ ○
Snacks	○ ○ ○

I am motivated because

Stuck to meal plan? ☐

Stuck to exercise plan? ☐

Calorie intake

I am:_____

Exercise Plan					
Activity	Time	Sets	Reps	Dist.	
					❏
					❏
					❏
					❏
					❏

Healthy & Happy Tasks

❏
❏
❏
❏
❏
❏
❏

Shopping List

❏
❏
❏
❏
❏

Today's 3 Positives

○

○

○

Notes

Bed Time:

Today's Step Count

Daily Plan & Tracker

Date:_____

Sleep: ◯◯◯◯◯◯◯◯

Water: ◯◯◯◯◯◯◯◯

Resting HR:_____

Today I feel

Wake up time:

Meal Plan		
Breakfast	◯ ◯ ◯	
Lunch	◯ ◯ ◯	
Dinner	◯ ◯ ◯	
Snacks	◯ ◯ ◯	

I am motivated because

Stuck to meal plan? ☐
Stuck to exercise plan? ☐

Calorie intake

I am:_____

Exercise Plan					
Activity	Time	Sets	Reps	Dist.	
					❏
					❏
					❏
					❏
					❏

Healthy & Happy Tasks

❏
❏
❏
❏
❏
❏
❏

Shopping List

❏
❏
❏
❏
❏

Today's 3 Positives

○
○
○

Notes

Today's Step Count

Bed Time:

Daily Plan & Tracker

Date:_____

Sleep: ⟨⟩⟨⟩⟨⟩⟨⟩⟨⟩⟨⟩⟨⟩

Water: ⟨⟩⟨⟩⟨⟩⟨⟩⟨⟩⟨⟩⟨⟩

Resting HR:_____

Today I feel

Wake up time:

Meal Plan

Breakfast	○ ○ ○
Lunch	○ ○ ○
Dinner	○ ○ ○
Snacks	○ ○ ○

I am motivated because

Stuck to meal plan? ☐

Stuck to exercise plan? ☐

Calorie intake

I am:_____

Exercise Plan

Activity	Time	Sets	Reps	Dist.	
					☐
					☐
					☐
					☐
					☐

Healthy & Happy Tasks

☐
☐
☐
☐
☐
☐
☐

Shopping List

☐
☐
☐
☐
☐

Today's 3 Positives

○
○
○

Notes

Today's Step Count

Bed Time:

Weekly Health & Fitness Tracker

Week of:_____

Sleep Goal:_____
Hydration Goal:_____
Calories Goal:_____

My Motivation

My Exercise Goal This Week

My Health Goal This Week

Words for When I Need a Motivation Boost

Exercise Log

	Goal	Actual
Mon		
Tues		
Wed		
Thurs		
Fri		
Sat		
Sun		

Positive thought:_____

Health Log			
	Sleep (hrs)	Water intake	Calorie intake
Mon			
Tues			
Wed			
Thurs			
Fri			
Sat			
Sun			

What Went Well?

Healthy Habits

Habit	M	T	W	T	F	S	S

Could Go Better

Next Week Will Bring

Daily Plan & Tracker

Date:_____

Sleep: ○○○○○○○○

Water: ○○○○○○○○

Resting HR:_____

Today I feel

Wake up time:

Meal Plan

Breakfast	○ ○ ○
Lunch	○ ○ ○
Dinner	○ ○ ○
Snacks	○ ○ ○

I am motivated because

Stuck to meal plan? ☐

Stuck to exercise plan? ☐

Calorie intake

I am:_____

Exercise Plan

Activity	Time	Sets	Reps	Dist.	
					❑
					❑
					❑
					❑
					❑

Healthy & Happy Tasks

❑
❑
❑
❑
❑
❑
❑

Shopping List

❑
❑
❑
❑
❑

Today's 3 Positives

○
○
○

Notes

Today's Step Count

Bed Time:

Daily Plan & Tracker

Date:_____

Sleep: ⬡⬡⬡⬡⬡⬡⬡⬡

Water: ⬡⬡⬡⬡⬡⬡⬡⬡

Resting HR:_____

Today I feel

Wake up time:

Meal Plan

Breakfast	○ ○ ○
Lunch	○ ○ ○
Dinner	○ ○ ○
Snacks	○ ○ ○

I am motivated because

Stuck to meal plan? ☐

Stuck to exercise plan? ☐

Calorie intake

I am:_____

Exercise Plan					
Activity	Time	Sets	Reps	Dist.	
					☐
					☐
					☐
					☐
					☐

Healthy & Happy Tasks

☐
☐
☐
☐
☐
☐
☐

Shopping List

☐
☐
☐
☐
☐

Today's 3 Positives

○
○
○

Notes

Today's Step Count

Bed Time:

Daily Plan & Tracker

Date:_____

Sleep: ◯◯◯◯◯◯◯◯

Water: ◯◯◯◯◯◯◯◯

Resting HR:_____

Today I feel

Wake up time:

Meal Plan

Breakfast	◯ ◯ ◯
Lunch	◯ ◯ ◯
Dinner	◯ ◯ ◯
Snacks	◯ ◯ ◯

I am motivated because

Stuck to meal plan? ☐

Stuck to exercise plan? ☐

Calorie intake

I am:_____

Exercise Plan

Activity	Time	Sets	Reps	Dist.	
					❑
					❑
					❑
					❑
					❑

Healthy & Happy Tasks

❑
❑
❑
❑
❑
❑
❑

Shopping List

❑
❑
❑
❑
❑

Today's 3 Positives

○
○
○

Notes

Bed Time:

Today's Step Count

Daily Plan & Tracker

Date:_____

Sleep: ○○○○○○○○

Water: ○○○○○○○○

Resting HR:_____

Today I feel

Wake up time:

Meal Plan

Breakfast	○ ○ ○
Lunch	○ ○ ○
Dinner	○ ○ ○
Snacks	○ ○ ○

I am motivated because

Stuck to meal plan? ☐

Stuck to exercise plan? ☐

Calorie intake

I am:_____

Exercise Plan

Activity	Time	Sets	Reps	Dist.	
					❑
					❑
					❑
					❑
					❑

Healthy & Happy Tasks

❑
❑
❑
❑
❑
❑
❑

Shopping List

❑
❑
❑
❑
❑

Today's 3 Positives

○
○
○

Notes

Today's Step Count

Bed Time:

Daily Plan & Tracker

Date:_____

Sleep: ⭕⭕⭕⭕⭕⭕⭕

Water: ⭕⭕⭕⭕⭕⭕⭕

Resting HR:_____

Today I feel

Wake up time:

Meal Plan

Breakfast	○ ○ ○
Lunch	○ ○ ○
Dinner	○ ○ ○
Snacks	○ ○ ○

I am motivated because

Stuck to meal plan? ☐

Stuck to exercise plan? ☐

Calorie intake

I am:_____

Exercise Plan

Activity	Time	Sets	Reps	Dist.	
					❑
					❑
					❑
					❑
					❑

Healthy & Happy Tasks

❑
❑
❑
❑
❑
❑
❑

Shopping List

❑
❑
❑
❑
❑

Today's 3 Positives

○
○
○

Notes

Today's Step Count

Bed Time:

Daily Plan & Tracker

Date:_____

Sleep: ⭕⭕⭕⭕⭕⭕⭕

Water: ⭕⭕⭕⭕⭕⭕⭕

Resting HR:_____

Today I feel

Wake up time:

Meal Plan

Breakfast	⭕ ⭕ ⭕
Lunch	⭕ ⭕ ⭕
Dinner	⭕ ⭕ ⭕
Snacks	⭕ ⭕ ⭕

I am motivated because

Stuck to meal plan? ☐

Stuck to exercise plan? ☐

Calorie intake

I am:_____

Exercise Plan

Activity	Time	Sets	Reps	Dist.	
					❑
					❑
					❑
					❑
					❑

Healthy & Happy Tasks

❑
❑
❑
❑
❑
❑
❑

Shopping List

❑
❑
❑
❑
❑

Today's 3 Positives

○
○
○

Notes

Today's Step Count

Bed Time:

Daily Plan & Tracker

Date:_____

Sleep: ○○○○○○○○

Water: ○○○○○○○○

Resting HR:_____

Today I feel

Wake up time:

Meal Plan

Breakfast	○
	○
	○

Lunch	○
	○
	○

Dinner	○
	○
	○

Snacks	○
	○
	○

I am motivated because

Stuck to meal plan? ☐

Stuck to exercise plan? ☐

Calorie intake

I am:_____

Exercise Plan

Activity	Time	Sets	Reps	Dist.	
					❏
					❏
					❏
					❏
					❏

Healthy & Happy Tasks

❏
❏
❏
❏
❏
❏
❏

Shopping List

❏
❏
❏
❏
❏

Today's 3 Positives

○
○
○

Notes

Today's Step Count

Bed Time:

Weekly Health & Fitness Tracker

Week of:_____

Sleep Goal:_____

Hydration Goal:_____

Calories Goal:_____

My Motivation

My Exercise Goal This Week

My Health Goal This Week

Words for When I Need a Motivation Boost

Exercise Log

	Goal	Actual
Mon		
Tues		
Wed		
Thurs		
Fri		
Sat		
Sun		

Positive thought:_____

Health Log

	Sleep (hrs)	Water intake	Calorie intake
Mon			
Tues			
Wed			
Thurs			
Fri			
Sat			
Sun			

What Went Well?

Healthy Habits

Habit	M	T	W	T	F	S	S

Could Go Better

Next Week Will Bring

Daily Plan & Tracker

Date:_____

Sleep: ○○○○○○○○

Water: ○○○○○○○○

Resting HR:_____

Today I feel

Wake up time:

Meal Plan

Breakfast	○
	○
	○
Lunch	○
	○
	○
Dinner	○
	○
	○
Snacks	○
	○
	○

I am motivated because

Stuck to meal plan? ☐

Stuck to exercise plan? ☐

Calorie intake

I am:_____

Exercise Plan					
Activity	Time	Sets	Reps	Dist.	
					❑
					❑
					❑
					❑
					❑

Healthy & Happy Tasks
❑
❑
❑
❑
❑
❑
❑

Shopping List
❑
❑
❑
❑
❑

Today's 3 Positives
○
○
○

Notes

Today's Step Count

Bed Time:

Daily Plan & Tracker

Date:_____

Sleep: ◯◯◯◯◯◯◯◯

Water: ◯◯◯◯◯◯◯◯

Resting HR:_____

Today I feel

Wake up time:

Meal Plan

Breakfast	◯
	◯
	◯
Lunch	◯
	◯
	◯
Dinner	◯
	◯
	◯
Snacks	◯
	◯
	◯

I am motivated because

Stuck to meal plan? ☐

Stuck to exercise plan? ☐

Calorie intake

I am:_____

Exercise Plan

Activity	Time	Sets	Reps	Dist.	
					☐
					☐
					☐
					☐
					☐

Healthy & Happy Tasks

☐
☐
☐
☐
☐
☐
☐

Shopping List

☐
☐
☐
☐
☐

Today's 3 Positives

○
○
○

Notes

Today's Step Count

Bed Time:

Daily Plan & Tracker

Date:_____

Sleep: ◯◯◯◯◯◯◯◯

Water: ◯◯◯◯◯◯◯◯

Resting HR:_____

Today I feel

Wake up time:

Meal Plan

Breakfast	◯ ◯ ◯
Lunch	◯ ◯ ◯
Dinner	◯ ◯ ◯
Snacks	◯ ◯ ◯

I am motivated because

Stuck to meal plan? ☐

Stuck to exercise plan? ☐

Calorie intake

I am:_____

Exercise Plan					
Activity	Time	Sets	Reps	Dist.	
					❑
					❑
					❑
					❑
					❑

Healthy & Happy Tasks

❑
❑
❑
❑
❑
❑
❑

Shopping List

❑
❑
❑
❑
❑

Today's 3 Positives

○
○
○

Notes

Today's Step Count

Bed Time:

Daily Plan & Tracker

Date:_____

Sleep: ⚬⚬⚬⚬⚬⚬⚬

Water: ⚬⚬⚬⚬⚬⚬⚬

Resting HR:_____

Today I feel

Wake up time:

Meal Plan

Breakfast	⚬ ⚬ ⚬
Lunch	⚬ ⚬ ⚬
Dinner	⚬ ⚬ ⚬
Snacks	⚬ ⚬ ⚬

I am motivated because

Stuck to meal plan? ☐

Stuck to exercise plan? ☐

Calorie intake

I am:_____

Exercise Plan

Activity	Time	Sets	Reps	Dist.	
					❏
					❏
					❏
					❏
					❏

Healthy & Happy Tasks

❏
❏
❏
❏
❏
❏
❏

Shopping List

❏
❏
❏
❏
❏

Today's 3 Positives

○
○
○

Notes

Today's Step Count

Bed Time:

Daily Plan & Tracker

Date:_____

Sleep: ○○○○○○○

Water: ○○○○○○○

Resting HR:_____

Today I feel

Wake up time: _____

Meal Plan

Breakfast	○ _____ ○ _____ ○ _____
Lunch	○ _____ ○ _____ ○ _____
Dinner	○ _____ ○ _____ ○ _____
Snacks	○ _____ ○ _____ ○ _____

I am motivated because

Stuck to meal plan? ☐

Stuck to exercise plan? ☐

Calorie intake

I am:_____

Exercise Plan

Activity	Time	Sets	Reps	Dist.	
					❑
					❑
					❑
					❑
					❑

Healthy & Happy Tasks

❑
❑
❑
❑
❑
❑
❑

Shopping List

❑
❑
❑
❑
❑

Today's 3 Positives

○
○
○

Notes

Today's Step Count

Bed Time:

Daily Plan & Tracker

Date:_____

Sleep: ○○○○○○○○

Water: ○○○○○○○○

Resting HR:_____

Today I feel

Wake up time:

Meal Plan

Breakfast	○ ○ ○
Lunch	○ ○ ○
Dinner	○ ○ ○
Snacks	○ ○ ○

I am motivated because

Stuck to meal plan? ☐

Stuck to exercise plan? ☐

Calorie intake

I am:_____

Exercise Plan

Activity	Time	Sets	Reps	Dist.	
					❑
					❑
					❑
					❑
					❑

Healthy & Happy Tasks

❑
❑
❑
❑
❑
❑
❑

Shopping List

❑
❑
❑
❑
❑

Today's 3 Positives

○
○
○

Notes

Today's Step Count

Bed Time:

Daily Plan & Tracker

Date:_____

Sleep: ⭕⭕⭕⭕⭕⭕⭕⭕

Water: ⭕⭕⭕⭕⭕⭕⭕⭕

Resting HR:_____

Today I feel

Wake up time:

Meal Plan

Breakfast	○ ○ ○
Lunch	○ ○ ○
Dinner	○ ○ ○
Snacks	○ ○ ○

I am motivated because

Stuck to meal plan? ☐

Stuck to exercise plan? ☐

Calorie intake

I am:_____

Exercise Plan

Activity	Time	Sets	Reps	Dist.	
					❑
					❑
					❑
					❑
					❑

Healthy & Happy Tasks

❑
❑
❑
❑
❑
❑
❑

Shopping List

❑
❑
❑
❑
❑

Today's 3 Positives

○
○
○

Notes

Today's Step Count

Bed Time:

www.ingramcontent.com/pod-product-compliance
Lightning Source LLC
Chambersburg PA
CBHW021604280526
45784CB00001BA/488